C000048681

SUPER FOOD

CUCUMBER

BLOOMSBURY

LONDON · OXFORD · NEW YORK · NEW DELHI · SYDNEY

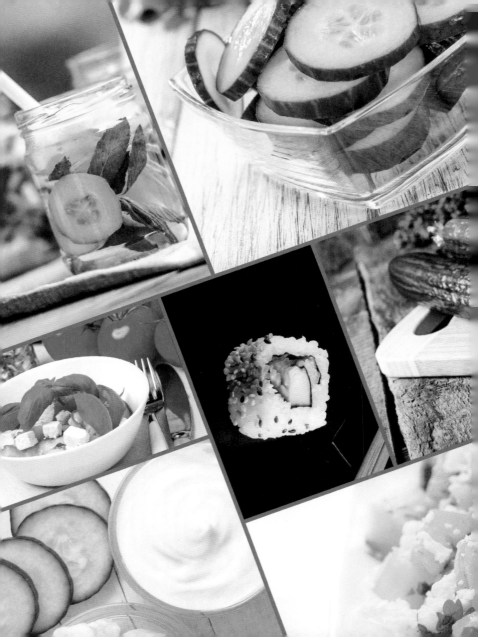

CONTENTS

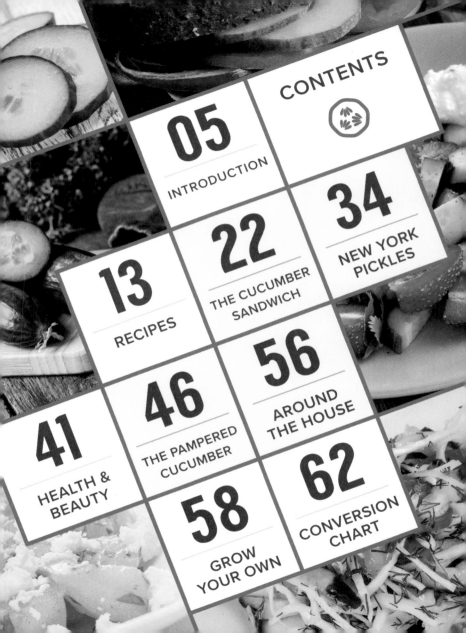

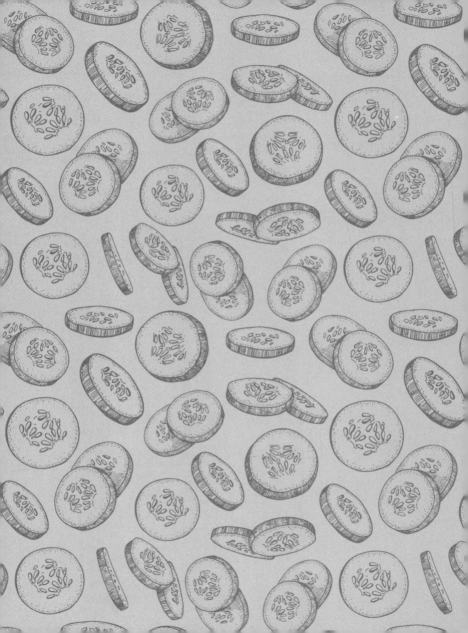

INTRODUCTION

'The prince enjoyed
exceptionally good health,
even for a prince; and owing
to his gymnastic exercises and
the scrupulous care he took
of himself ... he remained
as fresh as a great, green,
shiny Dutch cucumber.'

Leo Tolstoy, *Anna Karenina*
(1873–1877)

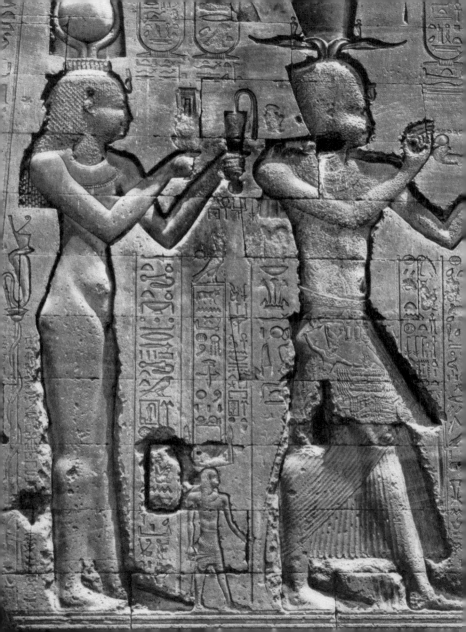

HISTORY

Millions of years ago in Asia a wild species of gourd flourished, the shared ancestor of both melons and cucumbers. It is believed the two strains diverged around 12 million years ago. Wild versions of cucumber were part of the diet of early man, and excavations at the Spirit Cave in Thailand have suggested that cucumbers were being eaten in the earliest Neolithic settlements.

The forerunner of our modern cucumber (*cucumis sativus*) is thought to have first been cultivated over 4,000 years ago in north-west India, and to have spread from there across the ancient world. The Israelites, fleeing with Moses, lamented in the Bible: 'O that we had meat to eat! We remember the fish we ate in Egypt for nothing, the cucumbers, the melon, the leeks, the onions and the garlic ...' (*Numbers* 11 v 5–6).

Ancient societies had discovered that pickling cucumbers in brine or vinegar was a good way to preserve them, and archaeological evidence shows that the Egyptians were pickling cucumbers they had imported from India. The ancients understood the nutritional value of pickled vegetables, and it is said that Cleopatra attributed her beauty to including them in her diet, while Julius Caesar fed them to his troops to keep them healthy.

The Romans were huge consumers of the cucumber, especially the emperor Tiberius, who had his slaves wheel huge barrows full of cucumbers around to keep them in the sun so he could enjoy them every day. The ancient Greeks enjoyed cucumbers too, although

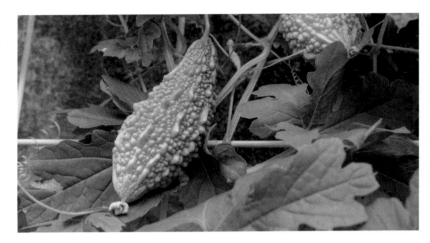

confusingly there was an archaic variety of melon which was cucumber-shaped and even tasted of cucumber. References in ancient texts to *sikyon* could therefore refer to melons as much as to cucumber. Given the shared ancestor of melons and cucumbers this lack of distinction is perhaps not surprising.

By medieval times cucumbers were being eaten across Europe and in the 9th century appear on a list of required plants for the gardens of the Emperor Charlemagne in Aquitaine. Their popularity was greater in eastern Europe at this time and from the 10th century the Slavic population enjoyed cucumbers as a central part of their diet, especially in their pickled form.

Christopher Columbus bought the cucumber to the New World at the end of the 15th century, planting supplies in Haiti for pickling to ensure nutrition on board his ships. The cucumber was popular with settlers, and through the process of trading goods the native American tribes were introduced to it and began to include it in the crops they grew.

The popularity of the cucumber has risen and fallen over the centuries, as there were times when people felt uneasy at the thought of eating uncooked vegetables. In England in the 1600s the cucumber was regarded with suspicion, and given the nickname 'cowcumber' – some said because it was only fit for cows, although it is probably just

> It is said that Cleopatra attributed her beauty to including cucumbers in her diet.

a pronunciation variation. At one point it was even regarded with dread, and a 16th century proverb held that 'raw cucumber makes the churchyards prosperous'. For a few centuries the cucumber fell from grace and it is thought that it only began to be eaten again in England in the reign of Henry VIII because it was enjoyed by Catherine of Aragon.

The original version of the cucumber was nothing like the long green cucumber of today. A copperplate image from the late 18th century shows a plant with small bean-shaped fruits. The cucumber was bred into the common form over centuries and there are now two main types that we use – slicing and pickling. Some varieties of slicing cucumber are called burpless (so-called because it was believed cucumbers could give you gas!). The cucumber is now firmly established as an everyday part of our modern diet and, as its health benefits are understood more fully, is set to stay.

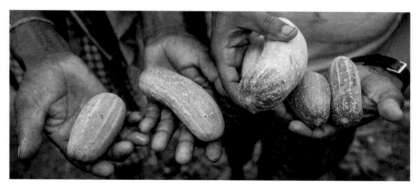

HEALTH BENEFITS

The unassuming cucumber packs a powerful punch when it comes to health benefits. With a staggering 96% water content, eating cucumbers to maintain hydration and flush out toxins has been popular for centuries, but the list of other, more impactful health benefits is truly impressive.

Cucumbers have incredible benefits for digestion. Although they contain virtually no calories, they do contain soluble fibre, which helps you feel full for longer. They also contain insoluble fibre, which is essential to good bowel health, and studies have shown that they also limit the body's ability to produce uric acid thereby reducing the risk of kidney stones.

Cucumbers are a great source of potassium and magnesium, which help with regulating blood pressure and combating stress. They contain a hormone that helps produce insulin and are therefore a good food for diabetics.

Eating cucumbers may also help reduce cholesterol thanks to high levels of sterols. They are also loaded with antioxidants including Vitamin C and beta-carotene, and polyphenols called lignans, which help fight cancer and heart disease. The skin and seeds of the cucumber contain the highest levels of Vitamin C. Their antioxidant properties also help inhibit inflammatory substances in the body and reduce pain.

Studies have demonstrated that cancer cell development can be inhibited by components in cucumbers called curcurbitacins. Curcurbitacins, which are found in other members of the gourd family, can be toxic if eaten in great quantities, and can give a slightly bitter taste to cucumbers. This is a defence mechanism of the plant against insects and herbivores. In cultivated cucumbers the bitterness

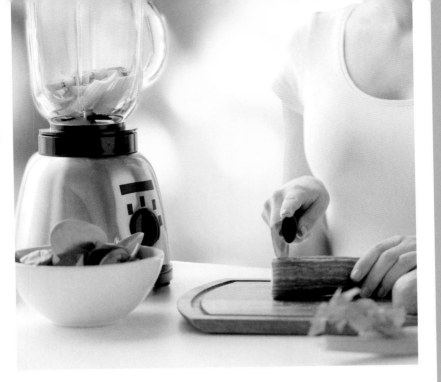

can be tackled by various methods during the growing process.

Cucumbers contain fisetin which helps with brain health by protecting nerve cells from the ageing process, thus fighting memory loss in conditions such as Alzheimer's. They also contain silica, an essential component of healthy tissue, which is great for skin and joints, and

Vitamin K, which is essential for bone health and calcium absorption. The Vitamin C in cucumbers also protects skin against UV rays, thus preventing wrinkles and other signs of ageing.

The cucumber – an immediate and easy source of nutrition and hydration – should be included in our diet every day!

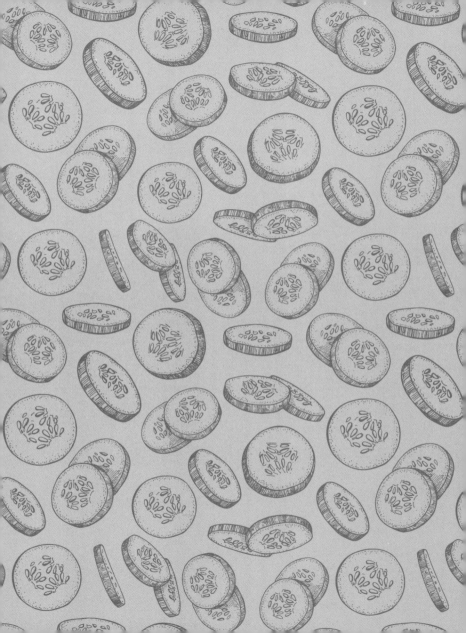

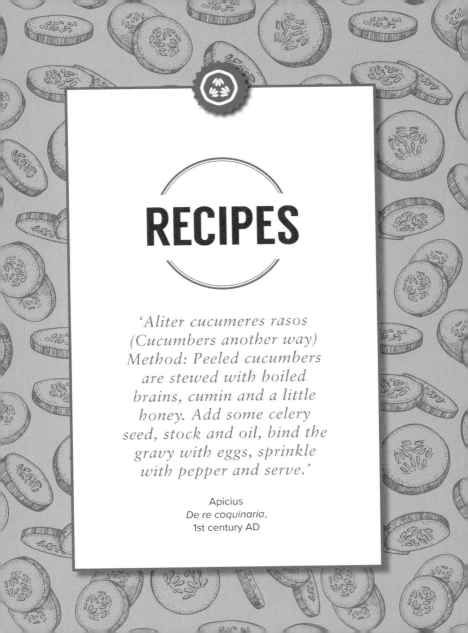

RECIPES

'Aliter cucumeres rasos (Cucumbers another way) Method: Peeled cucumbers are stewed with boiled brains, cumin and a little honey. Add some celery seed, stock and oil, bind the gravy with eggs, sprinkle with pepper and serve.'

Apicius
De re coquinaria,
1st century AD

SERVES: **2**
PREPARATION: **5 MINUTES**

BREAKFAST **SMOOTHIES**

Cucumbers are ideal for using in smoothies due to their high water content and mild flavour. Try these recipes for an instant energy boost to get your day off to a good start.

AVOCADO, SPINACH & APPLE

The calmness of the cucumber and avocado is given a kick with the addition of ginger and mint, while the apple juice adds sweetness. A great smoothie for cleansing the digestive system. Place all the ingredients in a blender and whizz until fully combined.

INGREDIENTS

- ½ cucumber
- ½ ripe avocado
- a small handful of spinach leaves
- 1 tbsp mint leaves
- a thumb-sized piece of ginger
- 200ml apple juice

MANGO & BANANA

Bananas contain potassium which is great for keeping you in a good mood, while mangoes are rich in Vitamin C and antioxidants. Blend all the ingredients together as above.

INGREDIENTS

- ½ cucumber
- 1 banana
- 100g mango chunks (you can use frozen ones)
- 100ml water

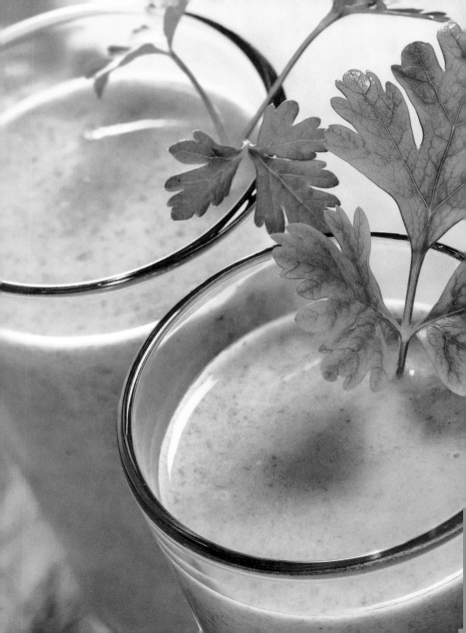

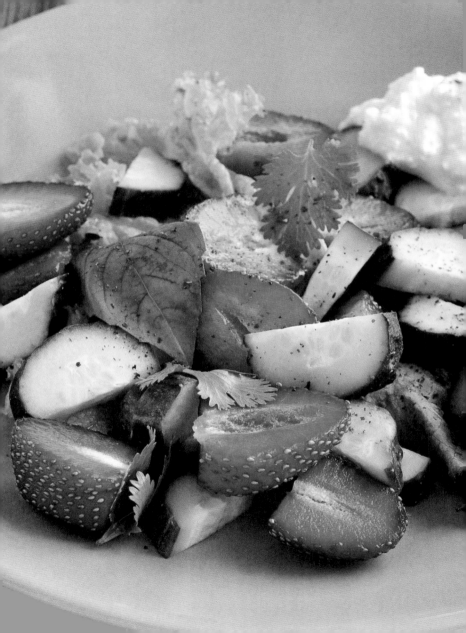

SERVES: 4
PREPARATION: 10 MINUTES

INGREDIENTS

- 1 cucumber
- 500g strawberries
- 4 tbsp extra virgin olive oil
- 2 tbsp balsamic vinegar
- 1 tsp honey
- salt and freshly ground black pepper
- baby leaf salad
- Greek yoghurt, to serve

STRAWBERRY & CUCUMBER SALAD

Strawberries and cucumber are a natural pairing for a delicious salad to keep you cool on a hot day. Add a dollop of Greek yoghurt to balance the tart flavours.

METHOD

Chop the cucumber and strawberries and place in a bowl. Combine the olive oil, balsamic vinegar and honey and season to taste. Serve on a bed of baby leaf salad accompanied by the Greek yoghurt.

RAILWAY ENGINEER GEORGE STEPHENSON, FRUSTRATED BY HIS BENDY CUCUMBERS, DESIGNED A GLASS CYLINDER TO ENCOURAGE THEM TO GROW STRAIGHT.

SERVES: 4
PREPARATION: 15 MINUTES

(GF) (V)

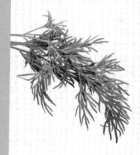

INGREDIENTS

- 2 cucumbers, sliced thinly
- small bunch of dill, chopped
- 2 tbsp sour cream
- 1 tsp cider vinegar
- ½ tsp sugar
- salt and freshly ground black pepper

POLISH SALAD 'MISERIA'

The name of this salad, meaning 'misery', is attributed to the homesickness of an Italian princess who in the 16th century married the Polish king Sigismund I and became Queen of Poland and Grand Duchess of Lithuania. Legend has it that whenever she ate this dish she wept for her native country. Alternatively it could be a reference to the miserable peasants who ate it because it was all they could afford!

METHOD

Place the cucumbers in a sieve, sprinkle with salt and leave for around ten minutes. Dry the cucumbers with kitchen towel, squeezing out any excess liquid. You can rinse the salt off completely if you like. Add most of the chopped dill to the cucumbers, retaining some for garnishing.

Mix together the sour cream, cider vinegar, sugar, salt and black pepper. Add the cucumber slices and toss together until the slices are coated, and chill for an hour. Garnish with the remaining chopped dill.

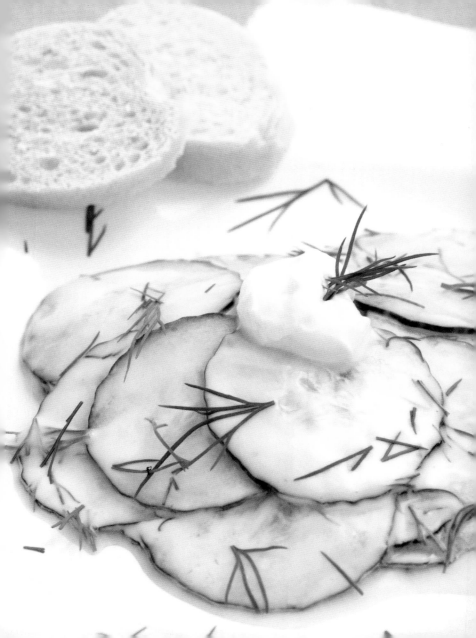

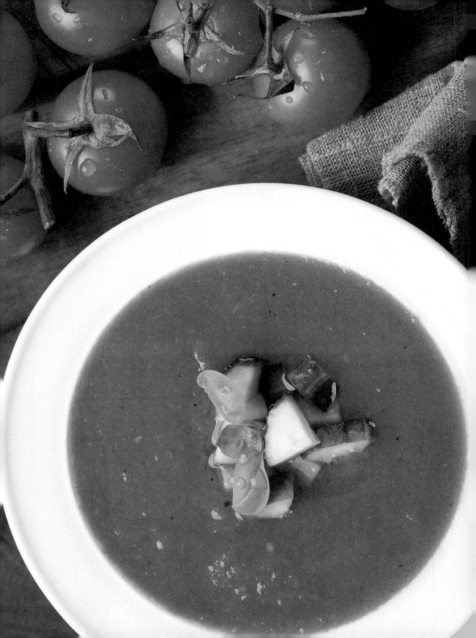

SERVES: 4-6
PREPARATION: 15 MINUTES

GAZPACHO

Gazpacho is a lovely cooling soup from Spain which does not need cooking, thus ensuring maximum nutrition value. Tomatoes, garlic and peppers add depth, colour and flavour.

INGREDIENTS

- 1 cucumber
- 450g ripe tomatoes
- 1 onion
- 1 red pepper
- 1 green pepper
- 400g tin chopped tomatoes
- 2 cloves garlic
- a slice of white bread, crust removed
- 2 tbsp sherry vinegar
- 6 tbsp olive oil
- a few drops of Tabasco sauce
- salt and freshly ground black pepper
- 200ml iced water

METHOD

Chop the vegetables and put a small amount of the cucumber to one side for the garnish.

Place all the vegetables into a food processor with the garlic and blend. Tear the bread into pieces and add to the mixture, together with the vinegar, olive oil, Tabasco sauce and seasoning. Pour in the iced water and blend until smooth.

Serve with the reserved cucumber scattered on top.

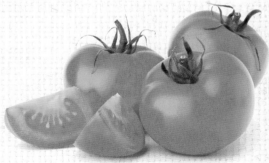

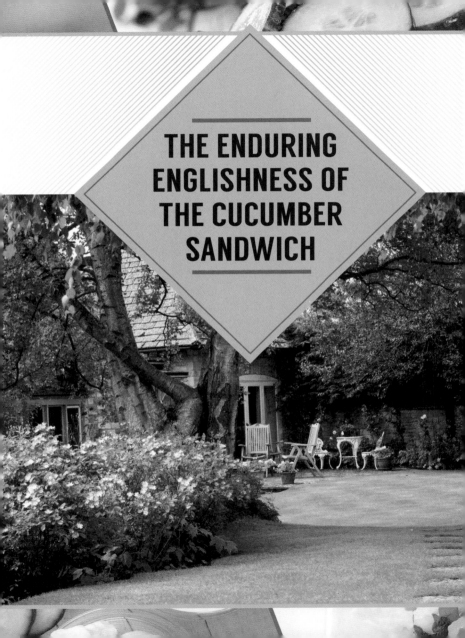

THE ENDURING ENGLISHNESS OF THE CUCUMBER SANDWICH

'... the shade of the cedar tree, the cucumber sandwich, the silver cream-jug, the English girl dressed in whatever English girls do wear for tennis ...'

Evelyn Waugh,
Brideshead Revisited, **1945**

The cucumber sandwich has come to epitomise the essence of Englishness, an image which was confirmed by Oscar Wilde in his 1895 play *The Importance of Being Earnest*, a light-hearted comedy of manners. The debonair bachelor Algernon's formidable aunt, Lady Bracknell, arrives for tea and naturally expects 'a cup of tea, and one of those nice cucumber sandwiches you promised me.' Sadly Algernon has eaten them all prior to her arrival whilst waiting with his friend Jack, who had commented on the sandwiches himself: 'Why cucumber sandwiches? Why such reckless extravagance in one so young?' Algernon's choice of cucumber sandwiches was an attempt to impress and to show his sophistication.

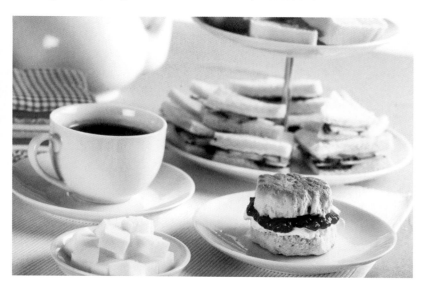

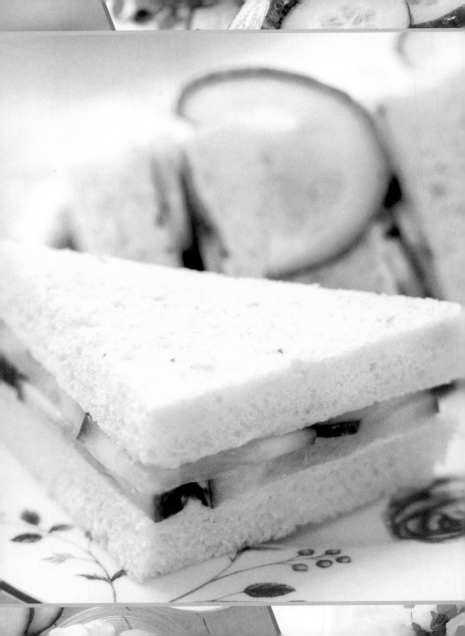

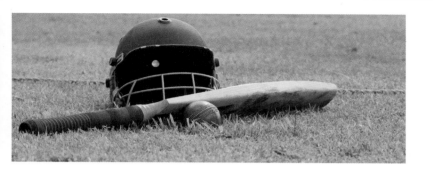

The Victorians invented the cucumber sandwich as part of afternoon tea or as a pre-dinner snack, and it reached its heyday in Edwardian England. As with Lady Bracknell, it was popular among the upper classes who could afford to eat food with little nutritional value: for this reason it was not popular with the working class. In addition, to consume cucumbers year-round they needed to be grown in greenhouses, a luxury that only the rich could afford.

When the British arrived in India in the 19th century they bought the cucumber sandwich with them – the cucumber had returned to its ancestral home! Adjusting to their new lives the colonials found a traditional afternoon tea with sandwiches ideal to help them keep cool in the unfamiliar heat, and they had the right idea. The cucumber's high water content helped avoid dehydration, while tea contains tannins which are a good cooling agent. Although it seems odd, hot drinks are better on a hot day as cold ones can shock an overheated system.

> *'Why cucumber sandwiches? Why such reckless extravagance in one so young?'*

Cucumber sandwiches, made with the thinnest possible soft white bread, crusts removed, are still an essential component of a traditional English afternoon tea, and are still served at tea time at cricket matches across the country, a quintessential part of that most British of sports.

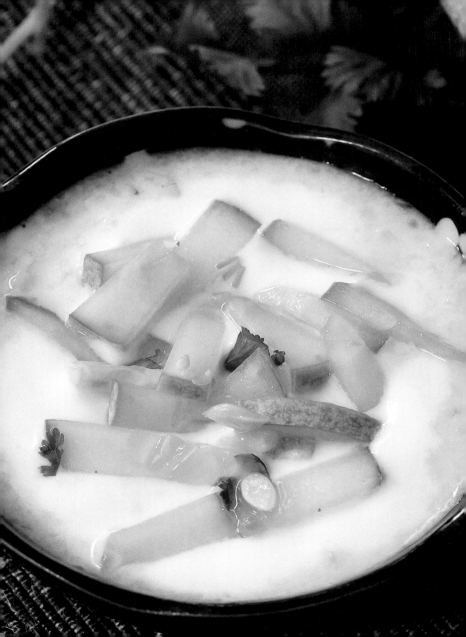

SERVES: 2
PREPARATION: 10 MINUTES

INDIAN
RATA

The cooling qualities of cucumber make it the ideal accompaniment for spicy dishes. This traditional dip combines cucumber with fresh mint and yoghurt, which also has a high water content, not to mention being loaded with healthy bacteria and protein.

INGREDIENTS

- ½ cucumber, peeled and finely chopped
- 300ml plain yoghurt
- 2 tbsp coriander leaves, chopped
- 1 tsp mint leaves, chopped
- 1 tsp ground coriander
- ½ tsp ground cumin
- salt and freshly ground black pepper

METHOD

Simply mix all the ingredients together in a bowl, chill and serve! This dish is ideal served with samosas, onion bhajis or any other Indian starters.

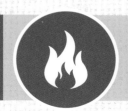

CUCUMBER HAS ALWAYS BEEN POPULAR IN HOT COUNTRIES DUE TO ITS HIGH WATER CONTENT. EATING SPICY FOOD ACTUALLY COOLS THE BODY DOWN TOO.

SERVES: 4
PREPARATION: 10 MINUTES

(DF) (VG) (V)

COUSCOUS & TOMATO SALAD

This simple refreshing salad is delicious served with grilled chicken or salmon as a light meal.

INGREDIENTS

- 150g couscous
- ½ cucumber
- 4 ripe tomatoes
- 1 clove garlic
- juice of ½ lemon
- 2 tbsp olive oil
- bunch of flat leaf parsley, chopped
- salt and freshly ground black pepper

METHOD

Place the couscous into a bowl and cover with boiling water so that it is completely covered with about 2cm extra to allow for expansion. Add ½ tbsp of the olive oil, cover and leave for about ten minutes or until all the water is absorbed and the couscous is soft.

Meanwhile chop the cucumber and tomatoes, crush the garlic clove and mix together with the lemon juice, olive oil and most of the parsley. Season to taste.

When the couscous is ready fluff it through with a fork. Add the cucumber mixture and scatter the remaining parsley leaves over the dish.

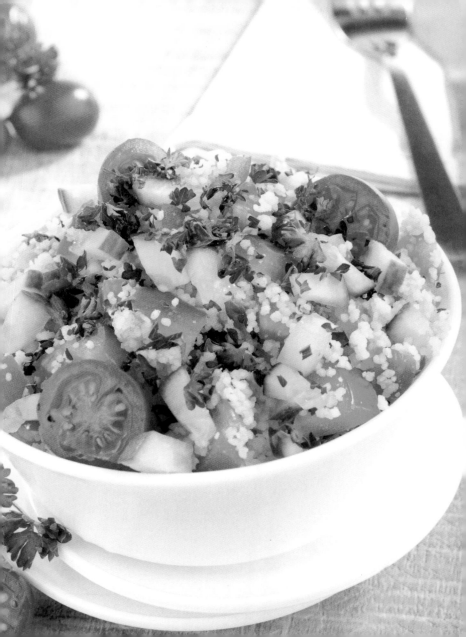

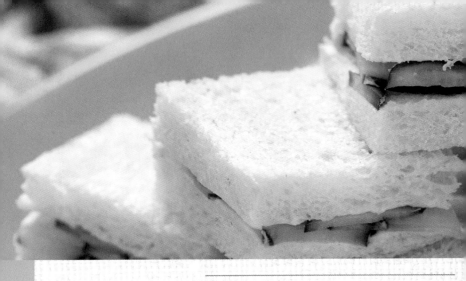

PERFECT
SANDWICH

SERVES: 2
PREPARATION: 5 MINUTES

The epitome of the English afternoon tea, the cucumber sandwich has come to evoke a gentler time gone by with its air of refinement.

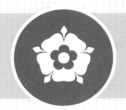

WHEN HENRY VIII'S WIFE JANE SEYMOUR WAS PREGNANT SHE CRAVED CUCUMBERS, WHICH HER STEP-DAUGHTER MARY TUDOR SUPPLIED FROM HER GARDEN.

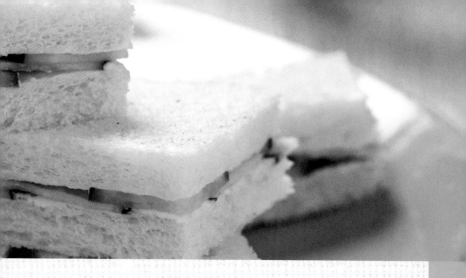

INGREDIENTS

- 4 slices of best quality thin white bread
- ½ cucumber
- butter
- salt and freshly ground black pepper
- juice of ½ lemon

 TOP TIP

For a variation on the classic recipe, you can replace the butter with cream cheese, or soak the cucumbers in vinegar for a traditional version.

METHOD

Trim the crusts off the bread with a very sharp knife to produce neat squares. Butter thinly to the very edges of the bread – this will prevent the damp cucumber making the bread soggy. Slice the cucumber finely and blot dry on a piece of kitchen towel before layering on to one piece of bread. Season with salt and freshly ground black pepper and a dash of lemon juice. Place the other piece of bread on top and cut into four quarters, or, if you prefer, you can cut the sandwich diagonally to make four triangles.

Enjoy with freshly-made Darjeeling tea from a teapot, served in the thinnest bone china, preferably sitting in a rose-scented garden. Or watching the cricket on a summer's afternoon …

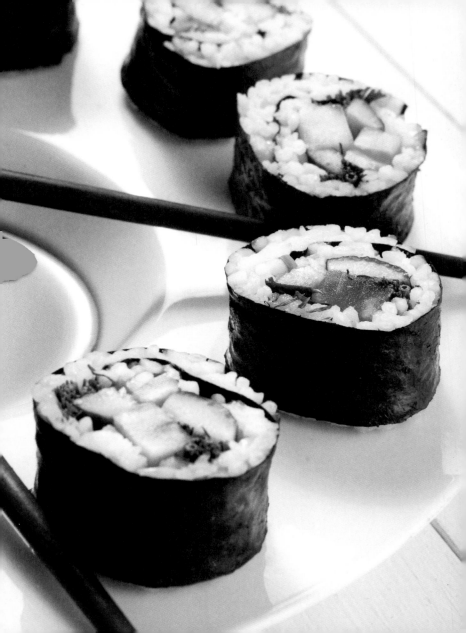

SERVES: 4
PREPARATION: 15 MINUTES

SUSHI
NORI MAKI

In Japan 'sushi' means a vinegar-flavoured cooked rice served with one or two simple ingredients. This recipe is 'nori maki', which means the sushi is served wrapped in rolls of seaweed.

INGREDIENTS

For the sushi:
- 250g Japanese sushi rice
- 1 tsp rice vinegar
- ½ cucumber
- 125g smoked salmon
- 4 sheets nori seaweed
- 2 spring onions, finely sliced
- soy sauce

For the dip:
- 1 red chilli
- 4 tbsp dark soy sauce

METHOD

Place the sushi rice in a pan of water with the rice vinegar, bring to the boil and simmer for around ten minutes. Drain well and allow the rice to cool while you prepare the other ingredients.

Cut the cucumber and salmon into long pieces. Lay the nori sheets on a sushi mat, or you could use a clean tea towel. Spoon a very thin layer of sushi rice over the sheet up to one edge, leaving a gap of a few cm at the opposite edge. Arrange the cucumber, spring onions and salmon along the middle, drizzle with soy sauce and roll up lengthwise so they are snugly held in the middle of the roll. Dampen the edges so they stick together, wrap in clingfilm and chill for 15 minutes or until firm.

Cut each roll crosswise into slices. To make the dip simply chop the chilli finely and add to the soy sauce.

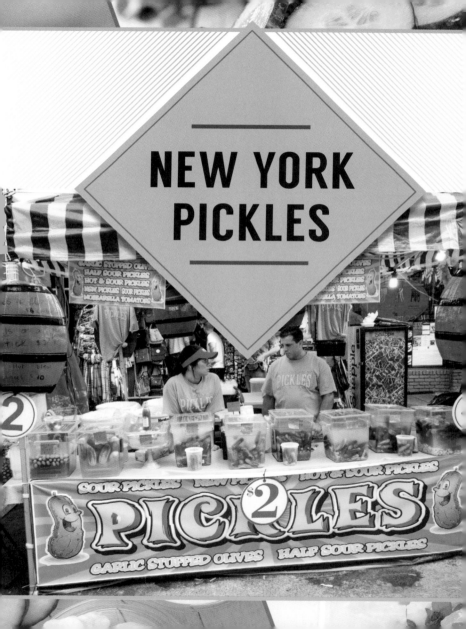

During the 17th century immigrant Dutch farmers arrived in the Brooklyn area of New York and planted and pickled vast amounts of cucumbers, creating the world's largest pickle industry.

Subsequent immigrants, homesick for the taste of their native countries, fuelled the huge demand for pickles. The Lower East Side Tenement museum website says that due to being 'available year-round, cheap, and ready to eat, pickles fed tenement dwellers and reminded many Eastern Europeans of the lands they had left behind'. The industry was also a great first source of employment for newly arrived immigrants who could cheaply rent a cart and sell street food. One such Jewish émigré, Izzy Guss, arrived in New York from Russia at the start of the 20th century and began selling pickles from a barrel in the area by then known as the Pickle District. By the time he opened his own shop in 1920 there were around 80 other pickle shops in the area. Although the pickle shops have nearly all gone now, the area maintains its connection with pickles with an annual Lower East Side Pickle Day.

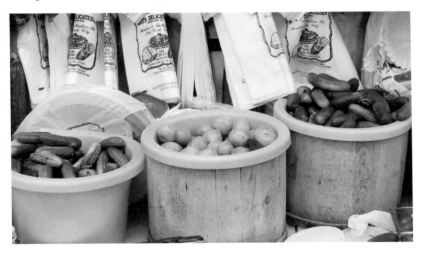

MAKES: 4 LOLLIES
PREPARATION: 15 MINUTES

ICE LOLLIES

The high water content of cucumber and melon makes them ideal for freezing in this recipe for a clean-tasting and healthy ice lolly.

INGREDIENTS

- 1 cucumber
- juice of ½ a lime
- 1 tbsp lime zest
- 160g melon chunks
- 1 tbsp agave syrup

METHOD

Blend all the ingredients and strain through a sieve. Pour the mixture into ice lolly holders, insert the lolly sticks and freeze overnight.

THE PHRASE 'COOL AS A CUCUMBER' WAS FIRST NOTED BY THE POET JOHN GAY IN HIS POEM 'A NEW SONG OF NEW SIMILES', WRITTEN AROUND 1715.

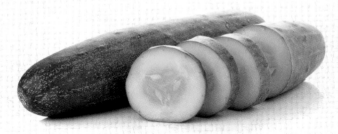

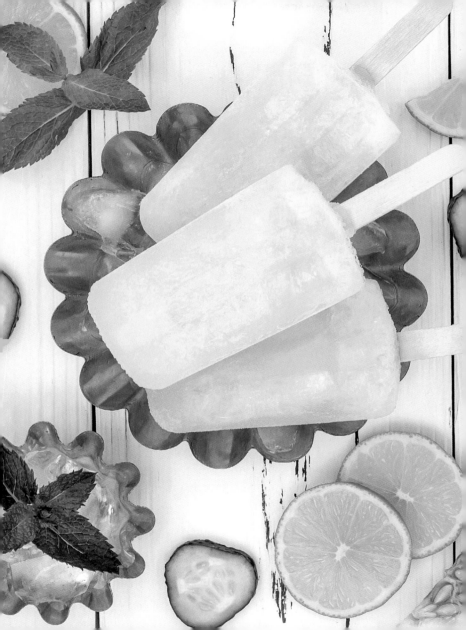

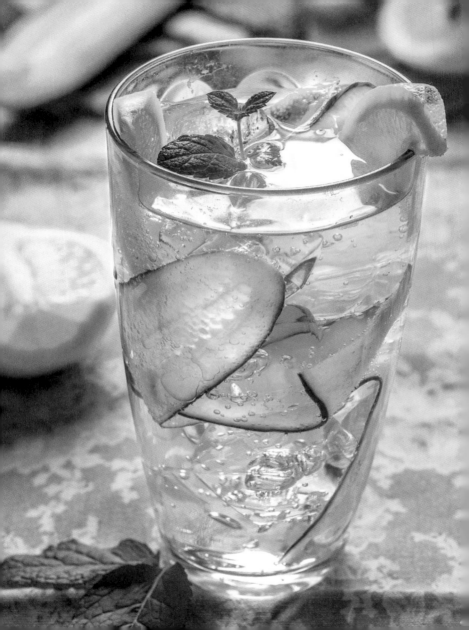

SERVES: 2
PREPARATION: 5 MINUTES

   (V)

GIN & CUCUMBER
COCKTAIL

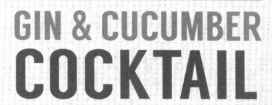

Try this light and refreshing twist on the classic gin and tonic.

INGREDIENTS

- ¼ cucumber
- ½ lemon, zest grated and juice squeezed
- 2 tbsp sugar
- 2 tbsp of mint leaves
- 60ml gin
- tonic water
- lemon slices, to garnish

METHOD

Chop the cucumber into slices and place in the bottom of the glasses, keeping some back for the garnish. Add the lemon zest, mint leaves, lemon juice and sugar and stir around to mix the ingredients. Add ice to the glasses and pour half the gin into each glass. Stir well and top up with tonic to taste.

Garnish with the remaining cucumber slices and lemon slices.

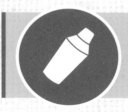

'JUICETAILS' ARE THE LATEST ARRIVAL IN FASHIONABLE BARS: CUCUMBERS AND OTHER VEGETABLES ARE COMBINED WITH TEQUILA. VODKA OR GIN TO CREATE 'CLEAN' COCKTAILS.

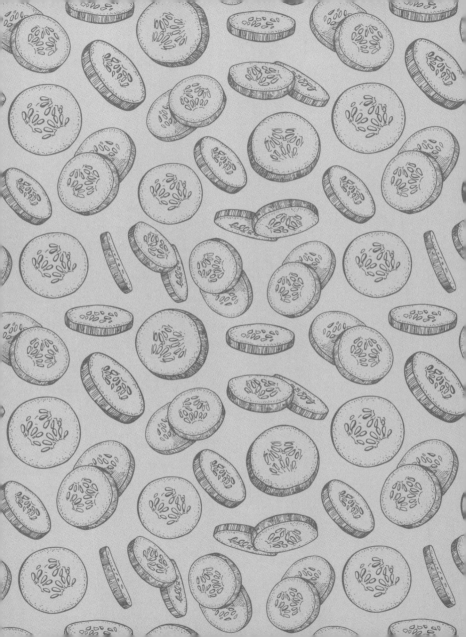

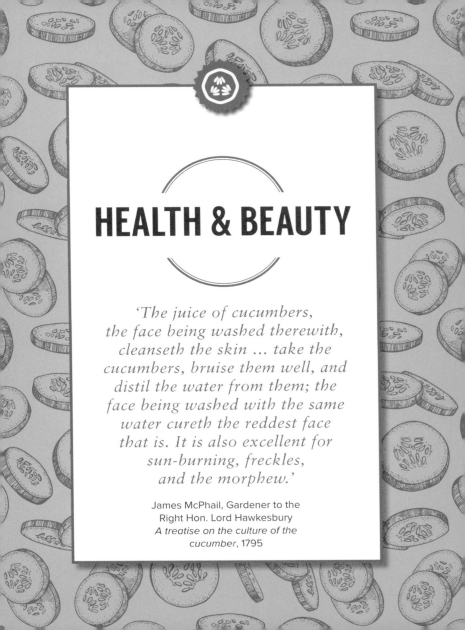

HEALTH & BEAUTY

'The juice of cucumbers, the face being washed therewith, cleanseth the skin ... take the cucumbers, bruise them well, and distil the water from them; the face being washed with the same water cureth the reddest face that is. It is also excellent for sun-burning, freckles, and the morphew.'

James McPhail, Gardener to the Right Hon. Lord Hawkesbury
A treatise on the culture of the cucumber, 1795

FACIAL TREATMENTS

Pamper your skin with these two facial treatments. While you relax place two slices of cucumber on your eyes to revive the eye area and reduce under-eye circles.

INGREDIENTS

- 2.5cm chunk of cucumber
- 1 drop rosemary essential oil
- 1 egg white

ANTI-BLEMISH MASK

Cucumber is calming while rosemary is a super-effective antiseptic. You'll find the egg white will tauten on your face.

Whizz the cucumber in a blender until it becomes completely liquid, then add the drop of rosemary essential oil. Whisk the egg white until stiff, fold in the cucumber mixture and smooth over the face avoiding the eyes and mouth area. Rinse off after 15 minutes using a clean, damp washcloth.

INGREDIENTS

- ½ cucumber
- 100g natural yoghurt
- a handful of oats

YOGHURT MASK

Cucumber, in combination with natural yoghurt, creates a gentle exfoliating treatment. The lactic acid in the yoghurt is a natural exfoliate and the cooling combination with cucumber also helps treat sunburn and reduce redness.

Blitz half a peeled cucumber in a blender. Mix the cucumber paste with the yoghurt and add the oats.

Apply the mask to your face as above.

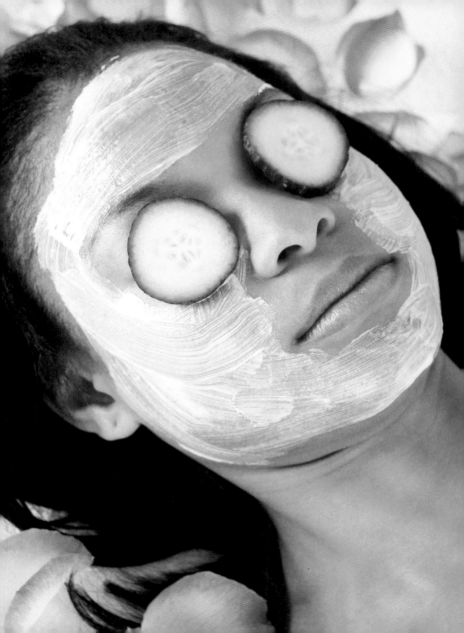

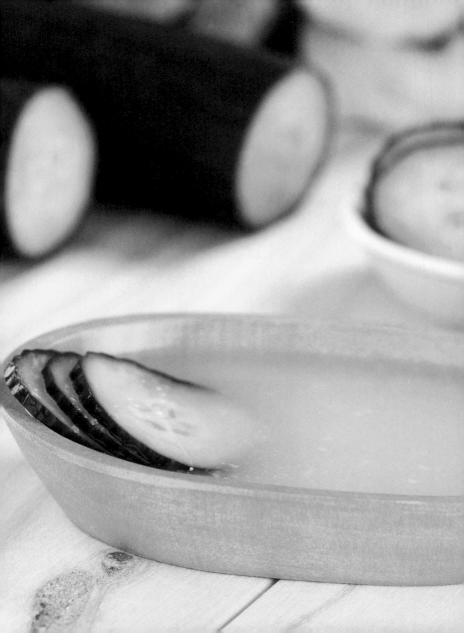

TONER

Cucumber has been a classic ingredient in toner for decades. With its great cooling properties, and natural oils to moisturise, it's easy to see why cucumber is such a firm beauty favourite.

 TOP TIP

Soak two cotton wool pads with the cucumber toner and place over your eyes to reduce puffiness.

METHOD

Take half a cucumber, peel and chop into small chunks (around ½cm each, or smaller if possible).

Place in a small saucepan and add 200ml water to cover the cucumber.

Bring to very gentle boil and simmer for around seven minutes – be very careful here to keep the heat low so you don't kill the nutrients. Leave to cool for around ten minutes before blending in a mixer until smooth.

Put the mixture through a sieve to strain out the pulp (discard the pulp but retain the water).

Pour the water into a clean, sterilised bottle and store in the fridge to be used as a refreshing toner once or twice a day after cleansing.

You can also pour a small amount into a travel-size spray bottle, for a refreshing spritz on the go.

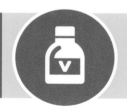 **THE VITAMIN C IN CUCUMBERS PROTECTS SKIN AGAINST UV RAYS THUS PREVENTING WRINKLES AND OTHER SIGNS OF AGEING.**

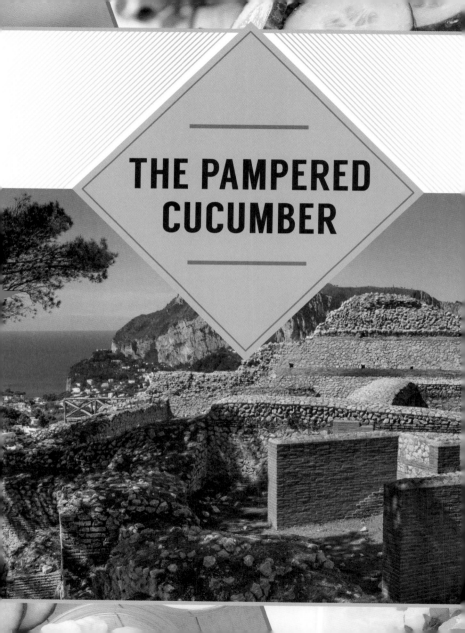

THE PAMPERED CUCUMBER

The need of an emperor for cucumbers led to the first greenhouse system. The cucumber was part of the diet of the ancient Romans, and the Emperor Tiberius (42 BC–37 AD) demanded cucumbers every day.

The Roman historian Pliny tells us in his *Natural History* that '[The cucumber] was a wonderful favourite with the Emperor Tiberius, and indeed, he was never without it; for he had raised beds made in frames upon wheels, by means of which the cucumbers were moved and exposed to the full heat of the sun; while, in winter, they were withdrawn, and placed under the protection of frames glazed with mirrorstone'.

The earliest greenhouse systems were known as specularia.

This passage describes one of the earliest greenhouse systems, known as the *specularia*. The Roman agricultural writer Columella explains the benefit of this, namely that by masking the cucumbers

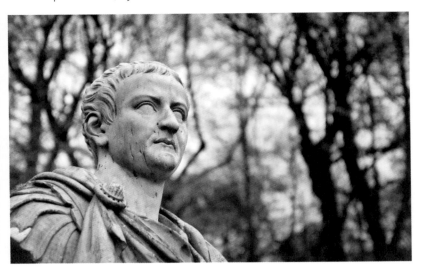

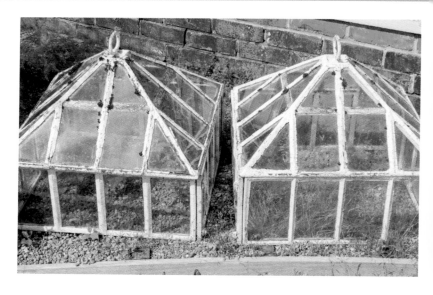

with see-through sheets '... even in the cold, on clear days, they can be taken out safe for the sun. By this method, cucumber was delivered to the Emperor Tiberius pretty well the year round.' The see-through sheets were made of a crystal called selenite, which the Romans called *lapis specularia*.

It is undoubtedly the case that the Romans would have continued to use this method to cultivate their vegetable and fruit crops; however, it seems that the idea of a glass-protected frame was not generally adopted in Europe until the 16th century. Early structures built for the protection of plants were sheds without windows, heated by such methods as placing hot embers in the floor, rather like the Roman hypocaust system.

In 1717 a design for a 'forcing-house' included a roof of glass, and from that time onward there were leaps forward in design, with ideas for style, method of heating and angles of roof glass. However, the window tax of 1696 and a glass tax of 1746 kept any experimentation with glass confined to the orangeries and hothouses of the very rich. With industrialisation the costs of making glass dropped, and greenhouse development really took off, with additions such as steam heating and structures made of iron instead of wood.

Gardening writers of the late 18th century and early 19th understood the challenges of cultivating cucumbers in the chilly British climate, and noted that in order to grow cucumbers 'the use of artificial heat with us is needful, to insure [sic] a successful growth.' The newly improved greenhouses were ideal for this popular crop.

Victorian conservatories became showcases for the aristocracy not only to display exotic fruits but to proclaim their wealth by access all year to such delicacies as the cucumber, enjoyed in their favourite sandwich. The wealthy aristocracy of Europe built more and more beautiful structures, one of the finest being the famous Palm House at Kew Gardens.

With a rising world population and demand for food, the need for intensive all-year-round farming has meant that greenhouses are today not just status symbols, but an essential part of food production. Britain's largest hydroponic greenhouse opened at Thanet in 2008 and each year grows, from January to November, around 13 million cucumbers!

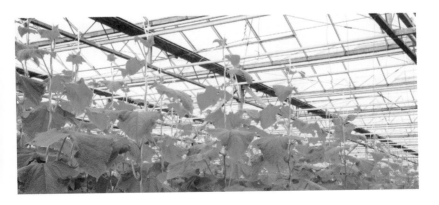

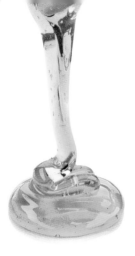

CELLULITE TREATMENT

Get rid of your 'orange peel' ... with cucumber! The dreaded cellulite affects people of all shapes and sizes and you can spend a small fortune on expensive treatments and lotions. Why not save your money and go for the natural remedy instead?

Cucumbers are rich in phytochemicals. When applied to the skin, they create a tautening of collagen, which tightens, firms and reduces the appearance of cellulite. Even better – in combination with other ingredients like coffee and honey – you can make your own home super-charged treatment to effectively smooth away your irksome lumps and bumps.

▼ TOP TIP

The caffeine in the coffee granules dilates the blood vessels in the skin, which tightens the surface. The caffeine also release toxins and metabolises fat under the surface.

INGREDIENTS

- 50g coffee granules
- 70ml cucumber juice
- 1 tbsp honey (preferably manuka)
- 1 tbsp granulated sugar

METHOD

Combine to make a paste-like mixture. Exfoliate the affected area with a dry brush, then apply the treatment and wrap in clingfilm to allow for maximum absorption. The natural warmth the film creates will help the nutrients soak in and do their work.

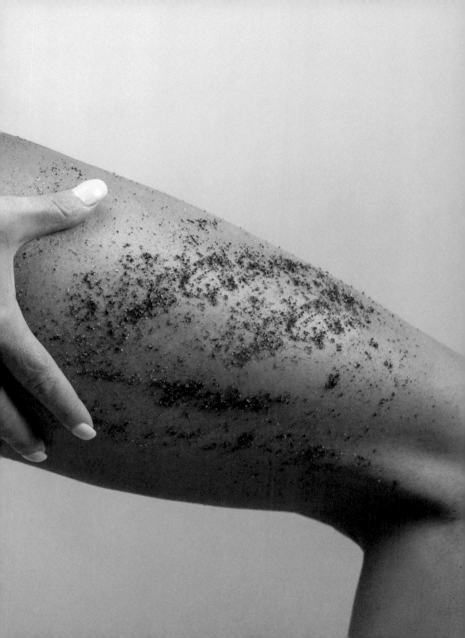

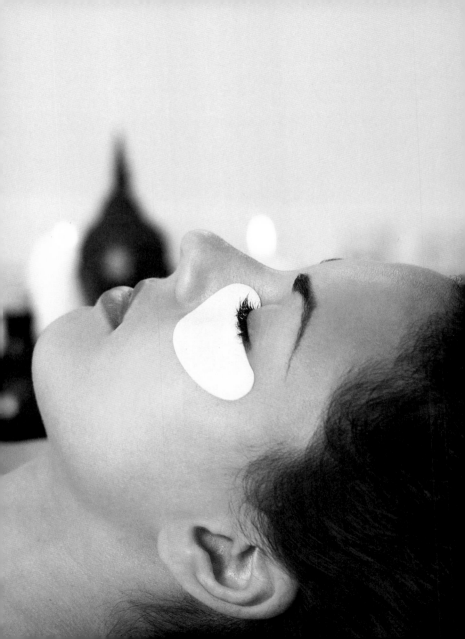

EYES

The image of sliced cucumber on the eyes is a classic, and with good reason. The ascorbic and caffeic acid in cucumbers reduces water retention, soothing puffiness and redness. Cucumbers also contain a very mild skin lightening property, which makes them a great treatment for dark under-eye circles.

METHOD

Blend cucumber in a mixer until you have a smooth paste. If you need to thin the mixture slightly, you can add small amounts of water, but go very carefully. When you have your mixture ready, soak the cotton pads in the liquid.

Carefully remove the pads and, keeping them flat, press them in your palms to remove excess liquid. The aim here is to keep them nicely saturated, but not soaking / dripping wet. Place the pads, flat, into freezer bags, and seal and freeze as quickly as possible to retain freshness.

Any time you need a refreshing ten-minute treatment, simply remove two pads from the freezer, allow to warm up for a couple of minutes, place over your eyes and relax.

TOP TIP

You can't help but relax while using this treatment, as you have to lie back and keep still to prevent the pads slipping off … the perfect excuse to take a break!

INGREDIENTS

- 1 large cucumber
- 15 cotton pads

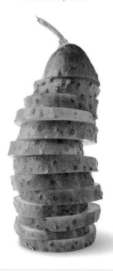

'SHAMPOOTHIE' HAIR TREATMENT

Cucumber contains Vitamins C, A, silica, and minerals such as potassium, magnesium and sodium, all of which promote healthy hair growth, repair and strengthening. Try this shampoo and conditioning treatment for hair and scalp.

METHOD

Blitz half a peeled cucumber in a blender. Add the lemon juice and oil and mix well.

Massage the paste into damp hair. For a more intense treatment, wrap your hair in a towel or in clingfilm. Leave for 15–20 minutes and rinse off with cool water.

INGREDIENTS

- ½ cucumber
- juice of 1 lemon
- ½ tsp olive, rosemary, tea tree or essential oil of your choice

 TOP TIP

You can apply and massage cucumber oil directly onto the scalp to aid hair loss, psoriasis and eczema.

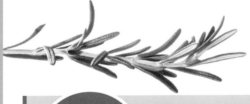

 **IN *NICHOLAS NICKLEBY* BY CHARLES DICKENS, NICHOLAS' MOTHER IS COURTED BY HER NEIGHBOUR WHO HAS BEEN THROWING CUCUMBERS OVER HER WALL TO ATTRACT HER!**

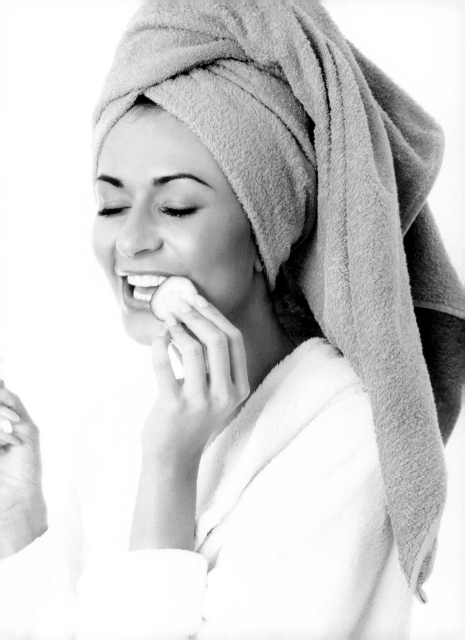

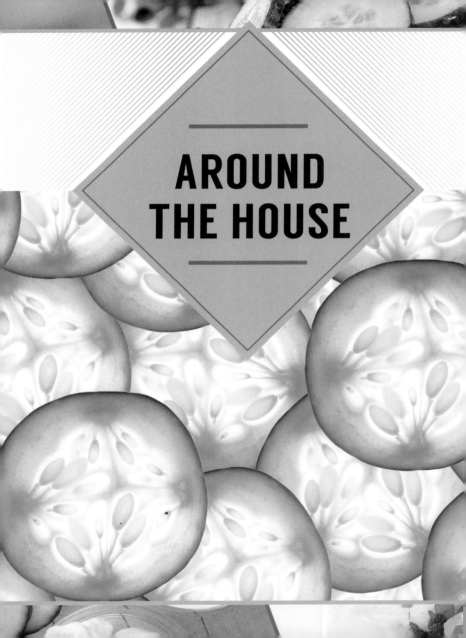

AROUND THE HOUSE

Is there anything the mighty cucumber can't do? There are many amazingly effective ways you can use it around the house.

Cucumber makes a superb cleaner for stainless steel. It can remove tarnish marks and bring back the shine in minutes. You can use it on sinks and taps for a brilliant lustre and it won't streak or stain. Just wipe around the area with a chunk of cucumber and rinse.

Dirty smudges and marks on walls (including those made by artistic children with crayon) can be quickly and effectively removed using cucumber, skin side, as an eraser.

Prevent your bathroom mirror from steaming up by rubbing the surface gently with slices of cucumber. The juice of the cucumber will then resist the damp air. It will make your bathroom smell lovely too!

You can use cucumbers to fix squeaky hinges. Simply rub the hinge with a slice of cucumber and the irritating noise will be gone!

You can even use cucumber as a shoe shine for leather shoes. Simply rub all over with a few slices of chunks of cucumber and wipe clean. This will provide not only great shine, but also repels water, making your shoes last longer.

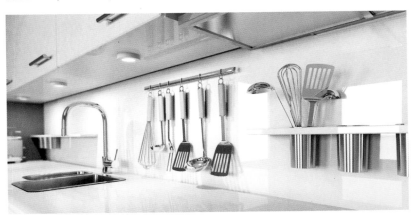

GROW YOUR OWN

Cucumbers are easy to grow, either in the ground, in growing bags or in pots.

Sow the seeds in early spring if you have a greenhouse or are planting indoors, or later if you are sowing outdoors to allow time for the soil to warm up. The seeds are large and flat so it's best if you sow them vertically so the new shoot can push its way out more easily.

Plant the seeds at a depth of around 2cm into seed compost, using biodegradeable pots if replanting to avoid root disturbance. Thin out the seedlings after a week or so, keeping the stronger ones.

If you are moving your seedlings outdoors allow them time to acclimatise to the colder conditions. Plant them into well-prepared soil mixed with a good compost. A horticultural fleece will help keep the soil warm if needed. Sow your seedlings in a sunny spot in rows 30cm apart.

You need to keep cucumber plants moist by regular watering as they have a shallow root system which can dry out. You must also support the baby plants as they grow, with garden canes or a vertical wire attached to the greenhouse roof.

Pinch out the growing point once it has reached the roof of the greenhouse, or if outdoors, after it has grown seven leaves, and after that pinch out side shoots with no flowers so the plant can direct its energy to growing cucumbers. It is advised that you feed your plants once a fortnight until the cucumbers appear, preferably using an organic, all-purpose fertilizer.

Harvest your cucumbers once they are big enough by cutting them with a sharp knife or garden secateurs. They should keep in the fridge for around a week.

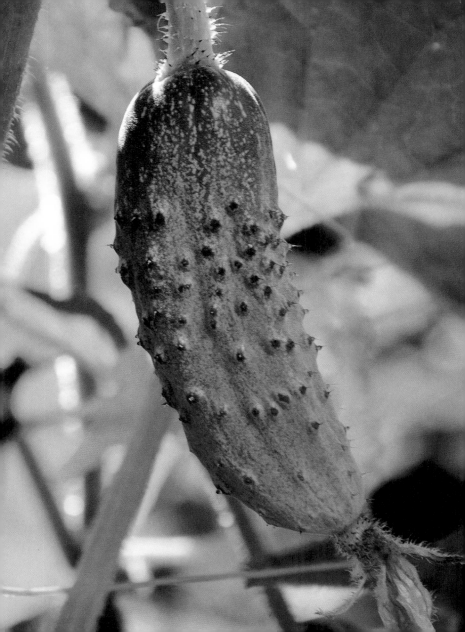

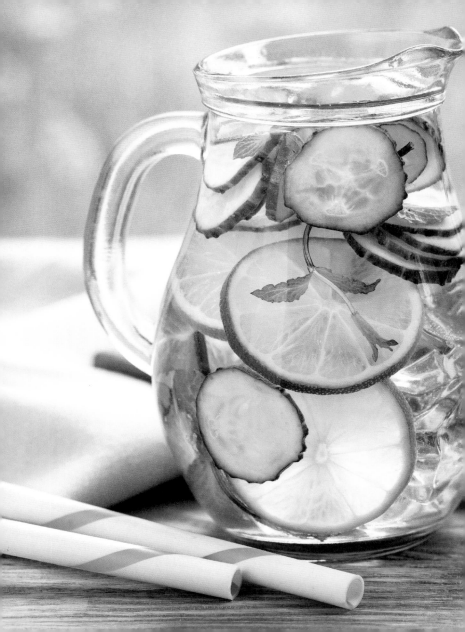

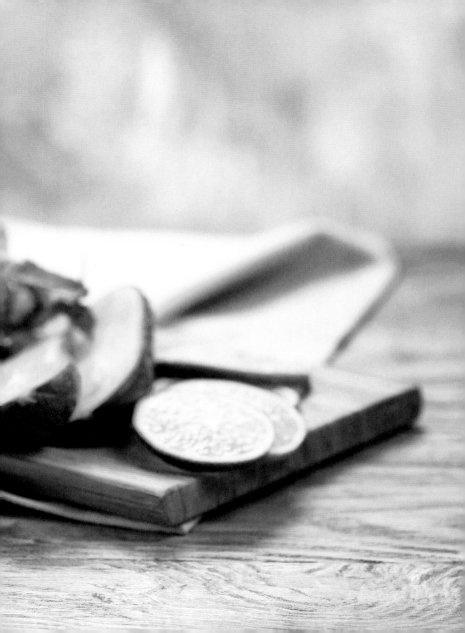

CONVERSION CHART FOR COMMON MEASUREMENTS

LIQUIDS

15 ml	½ fl oz
25 ml	1 fl oz
50 ml	2 fl oz
75 ml	3 fl oz
100 ml	3 ½ fl oz
125 ml	4 fl oz
150 ml	¼ pint
175 ml	6 fl oz
200 ml	7 fl oz
250 ml	8 fl oz
275 ml	9 fl oz
300 ml	½ pint
325 ml	11 fl oz
350 ml	12 fl oz
375 ml	13 fl oz
400 ml	14 fl oz
450 ml	¾ pint
475 ml	16 fl oz
500 ml	17 fl oz
575 ml	18 fl oz
600 ml	1 pint
750 ml	1 ¼ pints
900 ml	1 ½ pints
1 litre	1 ¾ pints
1.2 litres	2 pints
1.5 litres	2 ½ pints
1.8 litres	3 pints
2 litres	3 ½ pints
2.5 litres	4 pints
3.6 litres	6 pints

WEIGHTS

5 g	¼ oz
15 g	½ oz
20 g	¾ oz
25 g	1 oz
50 g	2 oz
75 g	3 oz
125 g	4 oz
150 g	5 oz
175 g	6 oz
200 g	7 oz
250 g	8 oz
275 g	9 oz
300 g	10 oz
325 g	11 oz
375 g	12 oz
400 g	13 oz
425 g	14 oz
475 g	15 oz
500 g	1 lb
625 g	1 ¼ lb
750 g	1 ½ lb
875 g	1 ¾ lb
1 kg	2 lb
1.25 kg	2 ½ lb
1.5 kg	3 lb
1.75 kg	3 ½ lb
2 kg	4 lb

OVEN TEMPERATURES

110°C .... (225°F) .... gas mark ¼
120°C .... (250°F) .... gas mark ½
140°C .... (275°F) .... gas mark 1
150°C .... (300°F) .... gas mark 2
160°C .... (325°F) .... gas mark 3
180°C .... (350°F) .... gas mark 4
190°C .... (375°F) .... gas mark 5
200°C .... (400°F) .... gas mark 6
220°C .... (425°F) .... gas mark 7
230°C .... (450°F) .... gas mark 8

MEASUREMENTS

5 mm .... ¼ inch
1 cm .... ½ inch
1.5 cm .... ¾ inch
2.5 cm .... 1 inch
5 cm .... 2 inches
7 cm .... 3 inches
10 cm .... 4 inches
12 cm .... 5 inches
15 cm .... 6 inches
18 cm .... 7 inches
20 cm .... 8 inches
23 cm .... 9 inches
25 cm .... 10 inches
28 cm .... 11 inches
30 cm .... 12 inches
33 cm .... 13 inches

KEY TO SYMBOLS

(DF) Dairy free

(GF) Gluten free

(V) Vegetariang

(VG) Vegan

A NOTE ON USING DIFFERENT OVENS

Not all ovens are the same, and the more cooking you do the better you will get to know yours. If a recipe says that you need to bake something for ten minutes or until golden brown, use your judgment as to whether it needs a few extra minutes. Conversely don't overcook food by following the timings rigidly if you think it looks ready.

As a general rule gas ovens have more uneven heat distribution so the top of the oven may be hotter than the bottom. Electric ovens tend to maintain a regular temperature throughout and distribute heat more evenly, especially fan ovens.

All the recipes in this book have been tested in an electric oven with a fan. Recommended oven temperatures are provided for electric (Celsius and Fahrenheit), and gas. If you have a fan oven then lower the electric temperature by 20°.

Bloomsbury Publishing
An imprint of Bloomsbury Publishing plc

50 Bedford Square
London
WC1B 3DP
UK

1385 Broadway
New York
NY 10018
USA

www.bloomsbury.com

BLOOMSBURY and the Diana logo are trademarks of Bloomsbury Publishing Plc

First Published in 2017

© Bloomsbury Publishing plc

Created for Bloomsbury by Plum5 Ltd

Photographs and Illustrations © Shutterstock

All rights reserved. No part of this publication may be reproduced or transmitted in any form or
by any means, electronic or mechanical, including photocopying, recording, or any information
storage or retrieval system, without prior permission in writing from the publishers.

No responsibility for loss caused to any individual or organization acting on
or refraining from action as a result of the material in this publication can be accepted
by Bloomsbury or the author.

British Library Cataloguing-in-Publication Data

A catalogue record for this book is available from the British Library.

Library of Congress Cataloguing-in-Publication Data

A catalogue record for this book is available from the Library of Congress.

ISBN: 9781408887370

2 4 6 8 10 9 7 5 3 1

Printed in China by C&C Printing

To find out more about our authors and books visit www.bloomsbury.com.
Here you will find extracts, author interviews, details of forthcoming events
and the option to sign up for our newsletters.